The Dumbest Things Smart People Say to Folks with MS

by
Dee Kite, PhD

Note: To protect the privacy and confidentiality of the individuals who shared their stories, the names, circumstances and certain other content details were modified to ensure such protection.

In this book I do not dispense medical or psychological advice or prescribe the use of any technique as a form of treatment for physical, emotional or medical problems. My intent is to offer information to help you in your quest for a full, meaningful, intentional life living with MS or loving someone who lives with MS.

I gratefully acknowledge the many people who live with MS or love someone with MS who contributed to the creation of this book.

Also by
Dee Kite

Mastering the Art of Success
With coauthors Les Brown, Mark Victor
Hansen, Jack Canfield, et. al
In Press

What You're Putting Up With is Holding You Back.
5 Steps to the Freedom You're Waiting For!

The Ropes Freedom Workbook
Companion to:
What You're Putting up With is Holding You Back
5 Steps to the Freedom You're Waiting For!

The Bloodless Stigmata
A Novel

For the folks who live with MS, their friends and their families.

Contents

Prologue

Being diagnosed with MS is not simple. Many of us have symptoms years before we're diagnosed. I was twenty-nine, in grad school. One morning I woke up numb on the left side. In the infirmary a physician's assistant poked me with a pin, "Do you feel this? (no) This? (no) This? (no)." He finally gave up and sent me back to my apartment. No answers. The numbness subsided after a few weeks. I forgot about it and went on with my studies.

Then there was the *fatigue*. One evening as other students bustled to their night classes, I just sat on the couch. I wondered, "Do other 31-year-olds feel this bad?" Every night I felt like I had the worst flu ever. I was so so tired. Like the physician's assistant, doctor after doctor after doctor listened to me and sent me away without an answer.

Seven years after the numbness was long forgotten I was living a great life. I was a professor at a university, wore designer suits and had an office with a window. I was engaged to Scott, a guy who "got" me. We bought my dream house: high ceilings and wooden floors on a treelined street. We had a beautiful summer wedding in the mountains of North Carolina and honeymooned in a lighthouse on an island off the coast of Maine. On the honeymoon I kept thinking my glasses were dirty. Eventually I realized it wasn't my glasses. I was losing the sight in my right eye. Scott and I went to play tennis and I just dropped the racket. I couldn't see the ball.

When we got home, the optometrist sent me to the ophthalmologist who, after having me look at a bunch of flashing bright lights, diagnosed optic neuritis. He handed me a pamphlet and said, "No one knows why people get it and there's nothing I can do..."

But it wasn't just my eye. The whole right side of my face hurt, like I had the flu on one side of my head. I just felt awful. I had to find out what was wrong.

My primary care physician sent me to the ENT. The ENT sent me to the neurologist–using the back door approach. He couldn't fit me into the regular schedule, and apparently, they considered me an emergency, so it was off to the hospital. I still remember the sunrise when Scott drove me and how neither of us commented on its beauty.

Seven hours after check-in, the neurologist swept into the room with his metal clipboard. He proceeded to give me tests. "Roll your arms this way. Now that way. Stand on one foot. Put your finger on your nose. Lie down. I'm going to scrape the bottom of your foot with this plastic card…"

'Not bad!' I thought, 'Wow, I'm doing really well! I'll probably get an A on this one.'

He scribbled on his pad and asked, "Has anything ever happened that you couldn't explain?"

I sat straight. "Yeah." The numbness.

He snapped the clipboard shut. "When you rolled your arms? You never used your left arm. When I scraped your foot? You had a Babinski response: your toe pulled back instead of moving forward. You've got Multiple Sclerosis."

That was just the beginning. MSers aren't just diagnosed and set free. There are many clinically-tested, FDA-approved treatments for MS and its symptoms (to slow the progression, not cure the disease). My neurologist watches my progress with regular MRIs. She has an infusion suite in her office with a long row of recliners where MS patients sit for their IV treatments. The National Multiple Sclerosis Society sends emails and a monthly magazine updating me on the latest treatments and the progress of clinical trials. We are an informed group of patients.

An informed group of patients with an unpredictable disease. MS hits each one of us in a different manner. Consider the early progression of my case. I had two significant exacerbations, seven years apart. Suppose the Physician's Assistant in the infirmary had diagnosed MS and one of my classmates had suggested that I try the Martini cure (It worked for her friend). Imagine that I started with nightly cocktails and voila! my numbness disappeared. I was symptom-free. The Martini cure really worked! My classmate could tell the world how Martinis cured me of MS...

This is the problem. Since the timing of an MS exacerbation is unpredictable and different for every patient, we cannot make a leap from one anecdotal Martini to a cure. MS patients know this. Many friends, family and acquaintances do not, which probably explains why many feel the need to offer us advice, even when we didn't ask for it.

Forward
by Dee's Father, R. Hayman Kite

I picked up the phone never realizing my heart was about to break.

My little girl, now a grown married woman, choked on her words..."Daddy I have MS."

MS! I had a vague idea about Multiple Sclerosis but what exploded into my mind was that MS has no cure...no cure! No cure meant I could not take her in my arms, like so many times when she was a child, and tell her I would make everything alright. I was overwhelmed with helplessness.

It wasn't until I gained some composure that I began the questions. What treatment is available? Are you in pain? Have you tried this? That? What did that doctor say? Eventually I understood and accepted the truth. My Daughter had MS. She knew the prognosis and was under the best treatment plan available.

Something I didn't expect was the pervasive feeling of guilt. I ought to be able to do *something*. But I could do nothing until I faced reality and saw things as they were.

I think the origin of my guilt was not taking an honest look at the reality of my life and my daughter's life. When I made suggestions or asked questions, I was acting out of my pain. I was simply increasing her fears. And until she began this book I did not know the weight of each question, each suggestion, on my little girl.

Slowly I gained control of my grief and negative images of her future.

She said, "Daddy, live *your* life in the present, the life *you* want. Not one burdened with thoughts about *my* life with MS."

It wasn't until I listened to Dee that I was able to be a positive force in her life. It wasn't until I listened that I understood Dee had confronted one of the most devastating diseases we humans may suffer and turned it into an opportunity to make a positive difference in the lives of others.

This little book documents how the human spirit can and does prevail.

Introduction

Whatever words we utter should be chosen with care, for people will hear them and be influenced by them for good or ill.

Buddha

Gusts of wind lifted the green balloons and their orange ribbons toward the sky. Thousands of walkers organized into groups, their laughter riding on the wind. They would walk, run, limp with canes, or ride in wheelchairs all in the name of finding a cure for Multiple Sclerosis.

I had come, not as a walker, but as a Life Coach living with MS. Inside the AT&T Center I sat at my table, hoping to spread the word to people living with MS that I could help them. Almost immediately, Pam rushed over to my table. She grabbed a pamphlet, glanced at it and leaned across the table. Tears drew shiny lines down her cheeks. "My daughter has just been diagnosed with MS. What can I do? I'm so scared."

Later Diane, a small woman with long brown hair, appeared in front of my table. She bubbled over with her dilemma. "My sister has MS and is in denial. She won't eat the proper foods. What can I do?"

After the walk I packed up my table. Outside I chatted with the hungry and tired who were waiting for sausages rolled in crispy bread. A woman, Michelle, sat in a wheelchair. She grasped my arm, sorrow and fear aching from her wide green eyes. "How can I get my husband to understand what it's like to have MS? He doesn't get it."

As Shakespeare wrote, "Therein lies the rub." For most of us living with MS, our symptoms are completely invisible. How can anyone "get it?" Even Michelle's husband didn't get it, and his wife was *in a wheelchair.*

What I heard that day supported what I already knew...we're in a pickle. It's as though all of us with this invisible, incurable chronic disease are on the South Rim of the Grand Canyon while our friends, family and coworkers are perched on the North Rim.

We're on opposite sides of a **grand** canyon. A great divide. And no one has installed phone lines yet. Yet on both sides we desperately need lines of communication. Consider this book the first step toward building an unusual phone system. A system that communicates what we **don't** want to hear.

I asked hundreds of men and women living with MS about the worst comments or advice they had received. I had my own cache of comments *I* didn't like to hear, yet I was still shocked at what the husbands, wives, children, parents, friends, coworkers, bosses, employees, in-laws and acquaintances of other MS patients had said.

Reactions to the Dumb Things Smart People have said to MS patients varied. Some patients were angry and dismayed. Some felt unloved and misunderstood. Some were even amused. But in all cases <u>they did not want to hear any of the comments</u>.

As one patient put it, "We're not seeking advice or sympathy—just understanding and acceptance." Another patient was frustrated with the "helpful" advice from so many who knew nothing about the disease and had no interest in learning. He would have preferred it if no one had even brought up the subject of MS.

It's important to note that in some cases the comments were hurtful or offensive only in context. For example hearing, "You look so good!" can be positive, especially, as one woman pointed out, if she's going on a date.

On the other hand, if Julie just told her friend, Sue, that she's been diagnosed with MS and Sue says, "But you look so good!" Julie might perceive it as an accusation; that Sue thinks Julie's lying or was misdiagnosed...that she can't really be sick. And as one respondent said (because we've all heard how good we look), "What am I supposed to do with that?" Julie could launch into an explanation of the pain she's feeling, that she's about to head home for bed, that she's numb on one side, that it feels like nails are being hammered into her palms. She could say what one patient says, "That's nice, but I'm just not fine." Or should she, as another woman put it, maintain the facade? "Why thank you, I'm so glad I look good." It reminds me of the old *Saturday Night Live* skit where Billy Crystal's character, Fernando Lamas, said, "Don't be a schnook, it's not how you feel, it's how you look. And you look Maaah-velous!"

Most of the time, the things people say are meant to be kind and helpful. But to those living with MS, it is easy to interpret their comments differently.

How about the advice? The ideas of things to try (such as a special diet or exercise) are welcomed if they come from a medical professional or another patient. Hearing the ideas from someone who doesn't have or understand MS is annoying and even stressful. Most of us have a team of doctors who oversee our treatment. For those of us who choose to listen to our doctors, hearing from someone else about some "snake oil treatment" that cured a friend or a friend of a friend just adds a wiggling doubt. Maybe I *should* run out and buy some snake oil. Maybe I'm not doing everything I can. Maybe...

A chorus of MS patients is shouting, MAYBE NOT!! They're tired of the comments. Tired of the advice.

Don't worry if some of these comments sound like something you already said. We all say Dumb Things when we're feeling uncomfortable, confused or preoccupied.

I still cringe when I remember what I said a year ago. On the last day of an author's conference I stood on the elevator with two fellow authors. Sandy and I had become close friends and we only knew a little about Dave. As the elevator ascended, Dave told us why he seemed so glum. "After 24 years of marriage, with no warning, my wife left me. I've got nothing."

Still giddy with hope and optimism from the conference, I launched into telling Dave why he didn't need to feel so bad, that as a coach I knew exactly how to help him, etc. etc. etc. With each of my ideas, he wilted a little more.

It wasn't until I'd been researching and writing this book that I realized how I'd not only passed up a great opportunity to truly listen to Dave, but left him feeling worse by going on and on about what he needed to do. Because of this book I've become acutely aware of the Dumb Things I say or am about to say. Thankfully, more and more of these comments stay in my head.

If you have a friend, an acquaintance or a loved one with MS, may this book be your first "phone line" across the vast divide.

Deal Breakers

Handle them carefully, for words have more power than atom bombs.

Pearl Strachan Hurd

Deal Breakers put a screeching halt to any real conversation. Technically, everything listed in this book is a Deal Breaker. But let's use this small list to ease into the idea that often we say things to another person without considering how she'll interpret it.

You may be thinking, "Wait a minute. If you're going to tell me what *not* to say, then what *should* I say to my friend?"

Say nothing. Your friend needs you to listen. Author Sue Patton Thoele said, "Deep listening is miraculous for both listener and speaker. When someone receives us with open-hearted, non-judging, intensely interested listening, our spirits expand."

Give your friend the gift of deep listening with the 1, 2, 3: I Hear You Method.

1, 2, 3: I Hear You Method

1. **Attention** Put your full attention on the person talking to you. Communicate your attention through eye contact, open body language (don't hide behind crossed arms or turn your body away) and make supportive sounds such as "Hmmm" or "Uh huh."

2. **Verification** To "hear" effectively, make sure you've understood the message the sender intended. Ask questions such as:

    "Is this what you meant?"

    "Are you saying...?"

    "Do I hear...?"

    If necessary, rephrase what you think the message is and ask if you're correct. Here is an example where verification allows you to drill down to the true message:

    Sender: "My husband is a wreck!"

    You: "Are you angry with your husband?"

    Sender: "No, I'm hurt because..."

3. **Intention** Make it your intention to hear the
   message. Let go of assumptions. Be authentic
   and LISTEN!

Attention

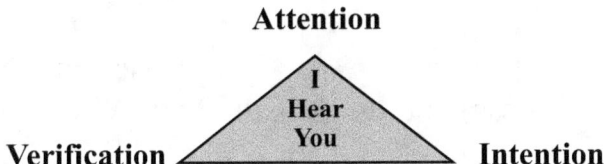

Verification **Intention**

Your friend just needs to be heard. She doesn't need you to moralize, offer advice, compare, play the authority or say any Dumb Things like:

You just have _____ (insert an illness) and don't really have MS because...you look so good!

God never gives you more than you can handle.

I can't deal with your issues.

Just ignore it.

You're too young to be so tired.

Don't sign up for the drug trial. If there was a real cure for MS, it would be in the news.

Well you didn't have to _____ (insert an activity). You could have let someone else do it.

MS just happens to some people.

I have that _____ (insert symptom), too. It happens as you get older.

Doctors have been known to be wrong, you know.

You're taking this so well.

Don't tell anyone you are in pain.

Get Over It

*If you wish to know the mind of a man,
listen to his words.*

Chinese Proverb

We've all seen the character...a drill sergeant, gym teacher, coach or other authority figure whose job is to turn weak-bellied recruits into champions. In movies or on television, the approach is consistent...verbal, emotional and physical abuse are the perfect recipe for turning out lean, mean, fighting machines or Olympic champions. In general, the more hateful this character, the more the recruits learn.

Sometimes this character isn't a person—it's a life-threatening trauma. In the movie version, the more the evil disease, accident or tragedy throws at the hero, the stronger she becomes. These familiar plots work great for dramatic purposes, but when we start to believe the Cinderella stories and act as if they're real, there are cruel, disheartening consequences.

The first consequence is the misguided, but honest belief that the sick among us should just get over our malady. The second consequence, also unintended but much more hurtful, is the implied message: being sick is a failure of inner spirit or the absence of a willingness to overcome.

Let's face it: living with MS creates enough drama on its own. The next time you see your friend with MS drooping a little bit, let go of the natural impulse to give him a "pick me up." The folks living with MS would like all drill sergeants in their lives to resign and refrain from saying:

It used to be a much bigger deal to have MS.

Keep taking it.

Suck it up.

Push through it.

You're strong. You'll get though this/be fine.

Ignore it and get on with your life.

Dust yourself off and get back in the saddle.

You shouldn't let it get you down.

There's nothing wrong with you.

Just try.

Put it in the back of your mind.

My _____ (insert person) has MS and s/he's doing just fine...climbs mountains...shows no symptoms...goes jogging every morning, etc.

That doesn't sound so bad.

Don't worry about not being able to _____ (insert an activity) anymore. Just let it go.

Why aren't you working more?

I can't believe you're still tired after that nap.

It's all in your head.

Who wouldn't be tired with that many kids?

You seem to be getting around just fine, so you ought to be able to _____ (insert activity).

You're not that sick.

You can still have a long, full life with MS.

At least you don't have the bad MS.

You're just not sleeping right.

It's not such a big deal to _____ (insert activity).

You won't die from MS.

An MS diagnosis doesn't mean what it used to years ago—they have so many more drugs to treat it.

If you would just try a little harder you could _____ (insert activity).

It's usually not a killer, so it can't be that bad, can it?

You have it, but it doesn't have you.

You should be grateful you don't have
_____ (insert a disease).

If things were that bad, you wouldn't be
sitting here.

You can still walk.

Maybe if you got another job you would
feel better.

Just Plain Mean

If you wouldn't write it and sign it, don't say it.

Earl Wilson

An MS diagnosis is like a boulder thrown onto the flat surface of a postcard-picture lake. Unlike a delightful dancing pebble skipping across the water, the MS boulder plunges deep into the lives of the patients and their families. Peaceful concentric ripples? No. More like a tsunami, crashing through relationships, hopes and dreams.

Intimate, long-term relationships are challenging enough without someone having a chronic, invisible (usually) disease. It takes thought, preparation and self-knowledge for all who face this wall of water to stand strong. Sometimes in the heat of an argument or when things seem hopeless, we crumble. Sometimes we forget the weight of our words:

John's mother died from MS.

You look too good to be on disability. Could I have your doctor's name, so I can get on it too?

I miss the old you.

What is wrong with you?

Since you are a Christian, you should be going around praising God instead of feeling sorry for yourself.

You don't know how to handle your MS. You get angry even though you knew that this _____(insert symptom) was going to happen to you. You have had it long enough to know better.

You have been sick for a long time. You don't need to keep talking about it just because you found out it's MS.

I get depressed when I talk to you.

You are in La La Land.

Come on, walk faster! We are tired of waiting for you.

I have my Christmas traditions and they don't include the food on your MS diet. Bring your own.

This is my friend, Jane, the one with MS. Jane, tell Suzy about your MS.

You're just being lazy.

These parking spots/motorized shopping carts are for the handicapped.

MS makes you impotent. What are you going to do when Jill wants it?

Stop playing the victim.

I sure hope she doesn't have that. All she needs is another excuse to be lazy. (an MS patient overheard this).

Oh God! What are you crying for?

You're giving in by using that cane. You're just a quitter.

A nurse told me that people with MS get really bad and end up being a burden on their family.

It's mind over matter.

You're going to be in a wheelchair and you won't be able to take care of your kids.

You're having intimacy problems? Tell your husband to masturbate.

Get used to the idea of being in a wheelchair.

You're the crippled one, right?

You've been able to do things you really *wanted* to do. I think you use MS as an excuse when you don't want to do something.

How come you used a wheelchair last week, but today you are just using a walker?

Quit work, go home, your life's over.

The Know-It-All Factor

I always advise people never to give advice.

P. G. Wodehouse

If you've ever practiced meditation, you know about the "monkey mind." We've all got it. Even if we try to sit still, our minds jump all over the place. "What will I buy George for his birthday? How can I finish that report before the deadline? That email is so funny. I need to make plans for the holidays. What is Congress doing now?"

Add a friend with MS into your monkey mind and it's bound to pop up like, "OMG, Diana has MS! She needs to do something! I've got to figure out how she can deal with this."

Often, because we're so burdened with the details of our own lives, we don't slow down to consider: "Does it seem like Diana needs or wants me to tell her what she should do about her disease?" When we pause to remember that folks living with MS work closely with their health care providers and have detailed treatment plans, it makes sense that they wouldn't want to hear what we think they should do.

I realize, as do others living with MS, it's difficult for someone who cares about us to watch us suffer without trying to do *something*. But you don't need to do anything. You can relax. Just *be* with us. Let us know you hear and understand the issues of our existence. Don't say:

You just have to get organized, then keep up with things on a daily basis.

Start taking better care of yourself.

You sleep too much. If you'd force yourself to stay awake, and if you'd get yourself out a little bit more, you'd feel so much better.

In a few years you are not going to have any of these "problems." Medical research will be so advanced that there will be a cure.

You just have to make yourself _____ (insert activity).

It's not MS. It's your age.

Stay positive and this thing will go away.

You can't possibly be that tired. Maybe you need different medications.

Have you ever thought about getting off the shots to see what happens?

Your legs might get stronger if you didn't use that cane all the time.

You don't really have to take a nap—just sleep in later.

You won't stagger or fall and your legs will be better if you go out every day for a walk.

No energy? Take a cold shower.

You shouldn't be riding. Get rid of those horses.

Get healthy and right and you will feel better.

The one thing you can control is your attitude, so have a good one!

Take a nap. You'll feel better.

You just have to retrain your brain and all
your symptoms will go away.

If you would go to church and believe,
you would be cured.

You really need to see people.
You HAVE to get out more.

Don't go to bed. You can stay up late and
sleep in tomorrow.

If you just concentrate your hands won't
shake.

Maybe you should talk to my friend
about what medicine she is on. It might
work for you.

Go to bed earlier, and you will not be so
tired.

My _____ (insert person) has MS and s/he was cured! You need to do what s/he did:

You should:
- Ride a horse
- Have all of your mercury fillings removed
- Walk more
- Take a cold shower
- Get into a closed container where they'll release hundreds of bees
- Go sit in a hyperbaric oxygen chamber
- Exercise more
- Get tested for Lyme Disease
- Get tested for Cat Scratch Fever
- Sleep on a metallic mattress pad
- Wear a magnetic bracelet
- Find God/go to church and believe you will be cured
- Explore Buddhism
- Explore Wicca

- Explore _____
  (insert speaker's religion
  of choice)
- Go to the chiropractor
- Go to the Holy Land and
  the Jordan River

You shouldn't:
- Walk so much
- Exercise so much
- Sleep so much
- Have kids
- Drive

You shouldn't eat:
- Sugar
- Wheat
- Gluten
- Microwaved foods
- So many vitamins
- Pork

You should eat or take:
- This special vitamin
  concoction
- A raw diet
- Royal Jelly

- More vitamins
- A better diet
- More vegetables
- _____(Insert Brand Name) Products
- A spoonful of honey sprinkled with cinnamon
- Special Chinese mushrooms
- _____(Insert MLM[1] Product)
- _____ hormones

You shouldn't drink:
- Diet drinks
- Alcohol

You should drink:
- _____ (Insert Brand Name) water
- _____ (Insert Brand Name) fruit drink
- _____ (Insert Brand Name) energy/healing drink

---

[1] Multi-Level Marketing

- Coffee
- More water to flush everything out—then go outside and run to sweat it off
- Green tea

The Blame Game

Do not judge and you will never be mistaken.

Jean Jacques Rousseau

It's comforting to think that the world is a fair place, that we all get exactly what we deserve. That way if we behave ourselves: eat right, exercise, follow the rules—we'll have a perfect life. This idea has been called the "Just World Hypothesis"[2]. In a "Just World" people have good lives because they've been good. People get sick because they've been bad.

I happen to know this isn't true because I'm perfect and the doctor still had the audacity to tell me I have MS. Seriously though, the idea of a fair world is deeply ingrained in many. It makes it easier to explain the terrible, the inconceivable and the unexplainable. If you can't *see* any of your friend's MS symptoms, it's hard to understand his suffering, much less to empathize. It's a lot easier to buy into the Just World Hypothesis: he just needs to do something different and he won't feel so bad. As with most invisible diseases, it's not true.

---

[2] Lerner, M. J. (1980). *The belief in a just world: A fundamental delusion.* New York: Plenum Press.

If you're ready to empathize and support your friend with MS, let go of the idea that the world is fair. Let go of the idea that looking good means feeling good. Let go of the blame. Don't say:

I think you can control this.

Why don't you want to _____ (insert activity) anymore?

You're a hypochondriac.

You are a pessimist. You'll make yourself better if you talk about the good of MS.

You must have some unrepented sin in your life.

You just have to learn to pace yourself.

You could work if you wanted to.

My _____ (insert person) has MS and is doing so much better than you.

If you just try harder, the MS will go away.

You don't look sick.

Just forget about it. I don't think you have it anyway.

My friend with MS doesn't act the way you do. She is always happy, no matter what happens to her.

I'm tired a lot and I can make it to functions. Why can't you?

Why do you have pain? _____ (insert person) has MS and is never in any pain.

I think if you tried harder, you could get past this.

You're just using MS as an excuse to be lazy.

Just Plain Clueless

The difference between the right word and the almost right word is the difference between lightning and the lightning bug.

Mark Twain

In a world where the discovery of new knowledge accelerates by the minute, being clueless is expected and accepted. There's just too much information to stay on top of everything that's happening. It's inevitable there will be something we don't understand. Inevitably we'll be clueless.

It's *not inevitable* that we'll forget to think before we speak. But there's a good chance it will happen. Let's face it—we've all been in the position where we wonder, "Why on earth did I say that?"

When it comes to being with a friend who has MS, it's okay to say nothing. It's okay not to have an "answer." Just try not to be clueless about your own cluelessness. Don't say:

_____ (insert person) has MS, so I know what you're talking about...I know just how you feel.

Oh, are you one of Jerry's Kids?

Is it an STD?

Are you drunk? (He was having trouble with his legs and had staggered).

I've decided that you don't have MS anymore.

Do you think if you lost some weight you would be able to walk?

Must be nice to sleep all day...I wish I could take naps.

Just quit your job. You work too much and it stresses you out.

Just how long are you going to have this?

MS does not cause pain.

Can my kids get it from you?

We all get tired.

Are you over that MS thing yet?

I didn't think MS could affect your brain.

I know what you mean about fatigue.
Sometimes I have to sit down to rest or
go take a nap.

How long do you have until you're in a
wheelchair?

Are you feeling less tired?

Stop! I told you not to do that.

Oh, I forget things all the time too.
Maybe I have MS.

Of everyone I know, you're the last
person I would expect to have MS.

You can't possibly have MS because
you're too old.

Your MS isn't that bad.

But you're too young.

But you can still get around okay.

There are just some symptoms that you're going to have to learn to live with.

The Smartest Things Smart People Say and Do

Kind words can be short and easy to speak but their echoes are endless.

Mother Theresa

By now you may be saying, "Alright already! I won't say any Dumb Things. And I'll use the 1,2,3 I Hear You Method. But it just doesn't seem like enough."

You're right. It's only *enough* when you take the time to truly understand your friend. Since each person is different, there isn't one right thing to say or do. Kate loves it when her friend says, "Don't make yourself tired" because she feels understood. But just because Kate likes it doesn't mean your fiercely independent friend, Jodi, won't get mad if you say, "Don't make yourself tired."

Carol likes it when, "Someone knows I am in bed and brings me lunch since I can't fix it! It makes me very happy that they think of me when I didn't even ask."

But guess what Joe wishes others would do for him? "Nothing. I just wish that they would interact and treat me as they did in the past. I'm still the same person inside that I was prior to becoming ill."

Most folks living with MS wish their family and friends would do three basic things:

1. Understand the disease and how it affects the MSer (remember it affects each of us differently).
2. Acknowledge how tough it is and how well the MSer is doing.
3. Figure out how to help and do it. Don't leave it up to the MSer to ask you. Many struggle with guilt, often feeling like they're an imposition.

Here are some Smart Things Smart People said to (or did for) folks with MS:

I can't even imagine how hard that must be.

I don't understand—teach me.

Only you know what helps.

Forty-seven years of MS and you are still working out? What an inspiration!

WOW! YOU ROCK! (after she told her story to a friend)

Stop trying to be so independent...I'm coming over tonight to do your laundry— no arguments!

Nothing. (Trish said, "I like it best when others simply treat me like an able-bodied person." Dave said, "I'd prefer if the subject of MS never came up.")

I'm sorry. Is there anything I can do to help you?

Tell me what you are feeling.

Will you let me help you do that?

I'm sorry you're stuck in bed and can't make it to the Christmas Party. Here's a plate of Christmas cookies and some coffee.

I know you can mow the yard, but I want to do it for you. It will take me only 10 minutes.

What does it feel like to live with MS?

I can tell you are tired. Why don't you sit down and I'll do _____ (insert task)?

36

I know you can _____ (insert task),
but if I'm here, so you don't have to.

I love you no matter what.

I don't know how you manage all that.

Is there anything I can do for you today?

I'm sorry you're having an MS sick day.
I brought you a magazine and a smoothie
to cheer you up.

Do you want me to fly home? What can I
do? I'll do some research.

What happens during a relapse? How
often do you have relapses? What
happens between relapses?

You're a brave lady.

Sit down and RELAX!

Listen to your body. Only you know how
it feels.

Sorry you've having such a hard time. I
brought flowers to brighten your day.

What is MS, anyway? (she could tell
they were genuinely interested in the
answer and it made explaining
everything easier)

Listen to your body. Only you know how
it's feeling.

When would you like to go to church?
Don't worry, I'll get you there.

Oh wow! Can I do anything?

Let me know if you need help with the
baby.

I'm sorry you're not feeling well. Go rest
and I'll make dinner.

I can't imagine how you must feel or
what you go through, but let me know if
there is anything I can do to make it
easier on you.

Conclusion

Each difficult moment has the potential to open my eyes and open my heart.

Myla Kabat-Zinn

Newly diagnosed with MS in 1995, I lived in a constant state of panic and struggled just to maintain some semblance of normalcy. I remember the first advice I received. Trudy, a woman brimming with confidence and good cheer, presented me with a flowered "Get Well Soon" card.

She told me, "You may not be able to do much about MS, but you **can** have a positive attitude."

I taped the card to the wall in my office, hoping it might help. It did the opposite. Each time I looked at it, I felt so ashamed because no matter how hard I tried, my attitude was NOT positive. Physically I was pretty much okay, because being blind in one eye and feeling like I had the flu every afternoon were not going to kill me. Emotionally I was not okay. I didn't know what would happen next and I was scared. I'd sneak out of the bedroom at night so my brand new husband, Scott, wouldn't hear me cry.

At the same time that I was trying to make sense of it all, Scott was going through his own "newly diagnosed" journey. Everyone who knows and cares about a person living with MS also "lives with MS." Husbands and wives, mothers and fathers, sons and daughters...their hearts are broken, their lives forever changed.

Most try to be compassionate. But, MSers have learned the hard way (as you've read in this book), many aren't truly conscious of the words they use to "deal" with us. Some speak from a frustrated place of confusion or fear, grasping for some easy way to fix what is, at the moment, unfixable.

And like my experience with Trudy's card, sometimes the things Smart People say don't help—they hurt. During the course of this research I have been amazed at the magnitude and emotional impact of "helpful" comments.

A surprising and important result of my research was the validation it provided. My questions generated such passionate responses that I knew I wasn't alone with the shame, guilt and irritation I felt from some of the things Smart People said to me. Many patients commented on how good it felt to know we shared similar experiences.

I've been thrilled to find that MS friends and family are also interested in the topic. At a recent conference I told Meg, the woman sitting next to me, about the book. She bounced with enthusiasm. "My friend was just diagnosed! I wish I could get the book now! I have no idea what to say to her."

If you know someone with MS, I hope this book will help you be with her. Just relax and BE.

If you are living with MS, I hope you feel a little more connected to the rest of us who struggle with the same issues. You're not alone. Your friends and family are doing their best to help.

Good luck. My heart is with you.

About the Author

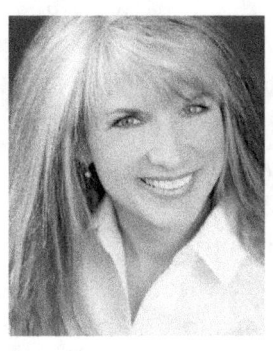

Dee Kite has lived with MS for more than 23 years. As a Personal Life Coach, she helps adults with MS thrive, not just survive. She is a speaker for the Lone Star Chapter of the National Multiple Sclerosis Society and is a former board member of the MS Center of South Texas. Her novel, "The Bloodless Stigmata," is an exciting murder mystery that gives the reader a behind-the-scenes look at the experience of being a professional woman diagnosed with MS.

With over 25 years experience in corporate, entrepreneurial and academic settings, Dr. Dee truly understands the various barriers anyone can face in their lives. She quickly and clearly enables her clients to identify obstacles and learn valuable take-away tools to work through life's toughest challenges to clarity, goal fulfillment and life success.

A sought-after public speaker and media guest, Dr. Dee imparts the wisdom she has gained from her own journey (as well as the experiences of the many she has helped) to teach and inspire others as they make their way in the world. Dee motivates people across America to take charge of their lives—and even have a little fun along the way—"It's always a good time to start!"

Dr. Dee has been interviewed by media around the world and speaks to groups across the country. She holds a PhD and an MBA. Her coach training is through CoachU the leading, internationally recognized institution for professional coaching. She is certified by the International Coach Federation and is a member of the San Antonio Professional Coaches Association.

Dee lives in San Antonio with her husband, Scott, and their two dogs, Trixie and Coconiña.

To learn more about Dee visit MyMSCoach.com or CoachKite.com.

Special Offer (Limited Time)

The Bloodless Stigmata

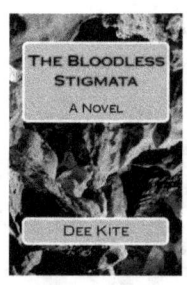

Dee's page-turning murder mystery, helps readers understand MS and how it can affect newly-diagnosed patients. It is a powerful tool for those who would like to understand the experience of their friends and family who live with MS.

Autographed Copy $12.95
(includes s&h)

Go to MyMSCoach.com/Special